PAMELA WOLFF

Strong Bones A Guide

Preventing Fractures and Maintaining Bone Health

Contents

I

"The world breaks everyone, and afterwards, some are strong at the broken places." - Ernest Hemingway

This book is the first in a series of books dedicated to bone health
and my beloved grandmother Josephine.
Stay-tuned for more titles by this author.

1

Introduction

Strong bones are the foundation of a healthy and active life. Yet, fractures and bone injuries can destroy this foundation, leading to pain, immobility, and a diminished quality of life. In this informational book, "Strong Bones: A Guide to Preventing Fractures and Maintaining Bone Health," we delve into the importance of bone health and provide practical strategies to safeguard your bones against fractures.

Understanding the fundamentals of bone health is crucial for everyone, regardless of age or lifestyle. By arming yourself with knowledge about bone structure, development, and the factors that contribute to fractures, you can take proactive steps to protect your bones and minimize the risk of injury.

Whether you're a young adult looking to build strong bones for the future, a middle-aged individual seeking to maintain bone density, or a senior aiming to prevent fractures, this book offers valuable insights and actionable advice. By adopting a holistic approach that encompasses nutrition, exercise, lifestyle modifications, and medical management, you can empower yourself to prioritize bone health and enjoy a life free from the limitations imposed by fractures.

Join us on this journey to stronger bones, improved mobility, and enhanced overall well-being. But first, who am I, the author of this guide? While I am not a medical professional, I have a personal history that has required me to educate myself in my bone health and the risks and opportunities there. Between the ages of 28 and 58, I suffered 5 fractures: both wrists, a foot, a shoulder and finally, my hip. I had no idea that my bone density could be an issue. I thought "This is just what happens to active people who engage in risky activities." For me, most of those fractures occurred while engaging in recreational sports like snow and water skiing, roller skating, and sled-riding. But finally, a simple fall in my home while playing with a new puppy sent me to the hospital for a fractured acetabular, or hip socket. It was in that moment, while lying helpless and alone on the floor and in pain, that I remembered my dear grandmother Jospehine. You see, Josephine was a vibrant and active octogenarian who tripped over a handbag which had been placed on the floor in her home and fractured her hip, an injury that would end her life less than a year after two surgeries. I worried if this was what was in store for me. I vowed in that moment to do whatever it took to understand my bone health, my risks and to reduce my chances of aging into infirmity. No thank you!

Along this journey, I have become a certified Functional Aging Specialist, a peer educator for American Bone Health, and a speaker and advocate for womens' health issues and owner of two OsteoStrong studios, a franchise dedicated to building and maintaining musculoskeletal strength. Musculoskeletal health is a highly important area of *everyone's* overall wellness; the importance of which, however, is not well communicated by our doctors or other medical professionals. It is my hope and purpose in writing this guide, to give you an easily followed and understood manual for developing, keeping or regaining strong bones.

As someone who has personally experienced the impact of fractures and bone-related complications, I understand the profound importance of raising awareness and sharing knowledge about bone health. Inspired by my own journey with osteoporosis and the devastating loss of my grandmother to a hip fracture, I am writing this book with a passionate commitment to empower others with the information they need to protect their bones and prevent fractures.

The purpose of this book is twofold:

1. **Raise Awareness:** By sharing my personal story and insights, I aim to raise awareness about the significance of bone health and the potential consequences of fractures. Many individuals may not realize the gravity of bone-related issues until they are directly affected or have a loved one impacted by fractures. Through education and awareness, we can highlight the importance of prioritizing bone health and encourage proactive measures to prevent fractures.
2. **Provide Knowledge and Guidance:** This book serves as a comprehensive guide to understanding bone health, identifying risk factors for fractures, and implementing effective strategies for prevention. Drawing upon scientific research, expert recommendations, and firsthand experiences, I aim to equip readers with the knowledge and tools they need to take control of their bone health and reduce their risk of fractures.

By sharing my personal journey, insights, and expertise, I hope to empower individuals, especially those who may be at higher risk due to conditions like osteoporosis, to prioritize their bone health and take proactive steps towards a future free from the burden of fractures. Together, we can raise awareness, build knowledge, and support one another on the path to stronger bones and improved well-being.

2

The Purpose and Function of Bones

The purpose of this chapter is to review the basics of bone health which encompass understanding the anatomy of bones, bone development, and strategies to maintain optimal bone density and strength. Bones are living tissues composed of collagen, calcium phosphate and calcium carbonate, and a dozen other minerals. They are not stiff, nor solid, but living, bending material that is both strong and flexible and able to withstand incredible amounts of stress or loading. In fact, loading or weight bearing actually stimulates bone growth as the bones respond to the stress by building more density and strength. Bones consist of a harder outer layer called cortical bone and a spongy and honeycombed interior called trabecular bone. It is said that the entire skeleton regenerates itself every 7-10 years.

Bones begin to grow in the womb and can be seen on ultrasound as early as 9 weeks with the mandible, scapula, clavicle and long bones ossifying by 12-16 weeks. The spine can be seen clearly in routine 20 week ultrasounds. Childhood and adolescence are critical periods for bone growth and development. During these stages, bones undergo rapid growth and increase in length, width, and density. Bone growth occurs primarily at the growth plates, which are areas of cartilage located near the ends of long bones. Hormones, particularly growth hormone and sex hormones (estrogen and testosterone), play key roles in regulating bone growth and development during puberty. Adequate nutrition, including sufficient intake of calcium, vitamin D, protein, and other essential nutrients, is crucial for supporting optimal bone growth and bone mineralization during childhood and adolescence

During this period, bones grow and increase in size rapidly through a process called bone remodeling, which involves the removal of old bone tissue by specialized cells called osteoclasts and the formation of new bone tissue by osteoblasts. This process is happening constantly as the cells in the bones turnover and rebuild; however as individuals age and particularly as hormone levels change during the aging process, there can be an imbalance in the process that allows more bone to be removed than what is rebuilt.

Peak bone mass occurs in early adulthood by age 30, with most or 99% of musculoskeletal development occurring by age 18 or 20. Women generally reach their peak sooner than men. Exercise and activity is usually enough to maintain bone density until about age 40, when most begin to lose bone mass, around 1% per year on average.

Bone Density and Strength

Throughout the book, we refer to bone density and strength, characteristics intimately connected to bone health. Bone density is the amount of mineral content in the bone tissue and is a key factor in determining bone strength. Bone mineral density or BMD measures the amount of minerals in the bone, primarily calcium and phosphorus. The more minerals in the bones, the denser and stronger the bones are and stronger bones are less likely to fracture. Optimal bone density and strength are essential in delivering those foundational benefits like supporting the body's weight, absorbing shock, and resisting fractures. Bone density is closely related to overall strength and physical function. Here's how:

- **Structural Support:** Bones provide structural support for the body, allowing us to stand, move, and perform daily activities. Bone density refers to the amount of mineral content in bone tissue, and denser bones are stronger and better able to withstand mechanical stress and load-bearing activities.
- **Resistance to Fractures:** Higher bone density is associated with greater bone strength and resilience, reducing the risk of fractures, particularly fragility fractures that occur with minimal trauma or force. Individuals with low bone density are more susceptible to fractures, which can lead to pain, disability, and limitations in mobility and function.
- **Muscle Attachment:** Bones serve as attachment sites for muscles, tendons, and ligaments, facilitating movement and providing leverage for muscle action. Stronger bones provide a more stable foundation for muscle attachment, enabling efficient muscle function and optimal physical performance.
- **Balance and Stability:** Bone density influences balance and stability, which are essential for maintaining posture, preventing falls, and avoiding injuries. Strong bones provide better support and stability, reducing the risk of falls and improving overall balance and coordination.
- **Joint Health:** Strong bones help maintain joint integrity and function by providing support and protection for the surrounding joint structures. Higher bone density can reduce the risk of joint degeneration and osteoarthritis, which can impair mobility and quality of

life.

- **Overall Strength and Function:** Strong bones contribute to overall physical strength and functional capacity, allowing individuals to engage in activities of daily living, participate in sports and recreational activities, and maintain independence and quality of life.

In summary, bone density is a critical determinant of bone strength and overall musculoskeletal health. Maintaining optimal bone density through proper nutrition, weight-bearing exercise, and lifestyle modifications is essential for promoting bone strength, preventing fractures, and preserving physical function and mobility throughout life.

Factors that Influence Bone Density

There are many factors that influence bone density and strength include genetics, nutrition, physical activity, hormonal balance, and lifestyle habits. All of these factors have a role to play in an individual's overall bone health and the way that individual will grow and age. It is important to consider these things over a lifetime and not just as a stopgap as one heads into the senior years. While improving habits and practices to promote better bone health is a worthwhile goal at any age.

While genetics play an important role, BMD (bone mineral density) and the risk of low bone density or diagnosed osteoporosis is impacted by the influence of several genes, not just one mutation of a single gene. Sometimes, just being aware of your family history is enough to help understand that part of your risk. Studies show that genetic factors are important in the development of bone density itself, as well as other inherited bio markers such as body mass index and the onset of menstruation and menopause. There may also be genetic factors that contribute to the structure and geometry of the bones themselves. What we do know is that while genetics plays a role, it is not the only important factor to consider. There are many other factors to consider, factors over which we have more control and opportunity to improve our risk factors.

Nutrition is everyone's starting point in building and maintaining healthy bones and it starts in childhood. Poor nutrition in childhood, particularly diets low in calcium and vitamin D, can sabotage a child's ability to grow to typical peak bone mass. Eating disorders during childhood or teen years can also cause malnutrition, negatively affecting their peak bone mass at a crucial time in a child's development. Bone loss due to anorexia nervosa can be seen in as little as 6 months and deficits can remain even after recovery. It has been suggested that achieving peak bone mass during these formative years can delay the onset of age related osteoporosis by as much as 13 years, further reducing the risk of fracture during the senior years when a fracture is most dangerous. Nutrition is not just for the young and plays a crucial role in maintaining a healthy foundation at all stages of life. During childhood and adolescence, however, much more bone is added to the skeleton than is removed, growing the bones and building density that can be impactful decades later. We will address nutrition with more detail, including foods that are rich in key vitamins and minerals a bit later in the book.

Calcium and vitamin D are essential nutrients for bone health throughout life. Calcium is required for bone mineralization and vitamin D facilitates calcium absorption and utilization. There are, however, other essentials for good bone health and these include vitamin k, magnesium, phosphorus and good quality protein. Other minerals with a key role to play include zinc which is required for bone mineralization and boron which aids the body in utilizing other minerals. Copper and iron play a role as do vitamins A, C, and all the B vitamins. It becomes easy to understand why overall good nutrition is so important, not just calcium intake. Another thing to consider is in recent years calcium supplementation has come under fire for causing kidney stones and colon polyps. Yet another study has linked calcium supplementation to calcium buildup in the arteries contributing to heart attacks and heart disease. The good news is that calcium is relatively easy to get in the diet, with planning and awareness of what foods are rich and easy to consume daily.

Physical activity is also an important part of maintaining or improving bone health. Physical activity in childhood improves bone mineralization and structure and lays a foundation of good skeletal health that may prevent osteoporosis in later life. Weight–bearing exercises, such as hiking, walking, running, dancing, and strength training, stimulate bone remodeling and help maintain bone density and strength at any age. Regular physical activity also improves balance, coordination, and muscle strength, reducing the risk of falls and fractures. New fitness technologies like OsteoStrong offer an easy and efficient solution to improving strength and many users have confirmed bone density improvements confirmed through x–ray scans called DEXA scans.

Lifestyle modifications are a third way to improve outcomes with regard to long–term bone health. Avoiding smoking and excessive alcohol consumption is important as these habits can negatively impact bone density and increase fracture risk. Smoking reduces blood supply to the bones and the nicotine slows production of osteoblasts, the bone building cells. Smoking also inhibits the body's ability to absorb calcium, which is necessary for many cellular functions in the body in addition to providing the foundation of strong bones. Additionally smokers take longer to heal from fractures. Smoking also causes inflammation throughout the body which contributes to conditions like osteoporosis among others.

Alcohol is known to increase cortisol, also called as the stress hormone, which decreases osteoblast production or bone building activity and increases osteoclast activity which contributes to further breakdown of bone. Alcohol abuse is also known to increase parathyroid hormone, an excess of which pulls calcium from the bones.

Finally, being aware of hormonal changes in the body is an action that can help you stay proactive in your bone health journey. Hormones such as estrogen, testosterone, growth hormone, and thyroid hormones regulate bone metabolism and influence bone density. Thyroid hormones are essential for bone remodeling and low or high levels can impact bone health in both children and adults. Estrogen is a great bone protector and stimulates osteoblast production throughout life. The sharp decline in estrogen during menopause is responsible for delivering many a shocking DEXA score, often to active women who thought they were in "good health". This was my story, despite my active sports related fractures, I felt I was fit and had been eating an organic, Mediterranean diet for years. I felt great, without aches or pain. But menopause is full of surprises, but we will try to stay focused on bone health

The Impact of Menopause

Menopause can have a significant impact on bone health due to the hormonal changes that occur during this transition. Statistically in the United States, one out of two women over 50 will break a bone due to low bone density. Menopause impacts every woman, so we will include some specific here on how menopause affects the bones:

- **Estrogen Decline:** During menopause, a woman's ovaries gradually produce less estrogen, leading to a decline in circulating estrogen levels. Estrogen plays a crucial role in maintaining bone density by inhibiting bone breakdown and promoting bone formation. The decrease in estrogen levels during menopause can accelerate bone loss, particularly in trabecular bone (spongy bone tissue), which is more responsive to hormonal changes.

- **Accelerated Bone Loss:** In the first few years after menopause, women may experience accelerated bone loss, with bone density declining at a faster rate than before menopause. This phase of rapid bone loss is known as postmenopausal osteoporosis and can increase the risk of fractures, especially in weight-bearing bones such as the spine, hips, and wrists.
- **Increased Fracture Risk:** The decline in bone density and strength during menopause increases the risk of fractures, particularly fragility fractures (fractures that occur with minimal trauma or force). Common sites for fractures in postmenopausal women include the vertebrae (spine), hip, and wrist.
- **Bone Remodeling Imbalance:** Estrogen deficiency alters the balance between bone resorption (breakdown) and bone formation, leading to increased bone turnover and a net loss of bone tissue. This imbalance in bone remodeling contributes to bone fragility and susceptibility to fractures.
- **Changes in Bone Structure:** Estrogen deficiency during menopause can also affect bone structure, leading to alterations in bone architecture and quality. Trabecular bone becomes more porous and less dense, while cortical bone (dense outer layer) may become thinner and more susceptible to fractures.
- **Other Factors:** In addition to estrogen decline, other factors associated with menopause, such as age-related muscle loss (sarcopenia), changes in body composition, and lifestyle factors (e.g., decreased physical activity, smoking, inadequate nutrition), can further exacerbate bone loss and increase fracture risk.

Overall, menopause represents a critical period of vulnerability for bone health in women, highlighting the importance of proactive measures to preserve bone density and reduce fracture risk. Lifestyle modifications, including weight-bearing exercise, adequate calcium and vitamin D intake, and avoidance of smoking and excessive alcohol consumption, are essential for maintaining bone health during and after menopause.

Another important part of managing bone health as we age is monitoring changes that may be occurring in the aging body. Osteoporosis is called the silent disease because it is often completely painless and symptom free until a fracture occurs. Knowing your risk factors, completing regular check-ups, and securing bone density tests can help monitor bone health and identify any abnormalities or deficiencies early on. DEXA, or dual-energy X-ray absorptiometry is a medical imaging test which has been considered the gold standard of bone testing and has been the primary tool used to diagnose osteoporosis since 1988. While guidelines for when to receive a DEXA scan vary, many women are not covered by insurance until age 65.

As with all medical interactions, advocate for yourself with your primary care physician if you have concerns about your bone density. If they are not responsive to your concerns, find another doctor. If that is not an option for you, find an outlet that offers ultrasound heel scans, generally offered for free at health fairs and corporate wellness events. While not a tool for diagnosis, it is a safe way to get feedback on your bone density in one area of the body and the machine produces a report that can be shared with your doctor

Additionally, healthcare providers may recommend bone density testing and, if necessary, pharmacological interventions to prevent or treat osteoporosis in postmenopausal women at high risk of fractures. A note of caution here however, traditional therapies for treating osteoporosis are often limited to pharmaceutical interventions and may not be the first solution individuals may want to try when faced with a diagnosis of osteoporosis and evaluating the potential of benefits over the potential side-effects. Changes to diet and exercise can be effective with dedication and understanding of the changes that may be necessary. Even if medication is determined to be the best route for an individual, the best solution includes looking at all areas that can be improved for better results.

That is one of the primary reasons for awareness and practices that support bone health from an early age as well as understanding the practices that support bone health in a holistic and natural way throughout a lifetime, practices without negative side effects and many long-term benefits.

Incorporating these basic principles of bone health into daily life: bone health supporting nutrition; weight bearing exercise; and living a healthy lifestyle free of smoking and alcohol abuse; is a good determinant of future bone health. Achieving optimal peak bone mass during adolescence and young adulthood is important for reducing the risk of osteoporosis and fractures later in life. Throughout life, bones undergo a continuous process of remodeling, where old bone tissue is resorbed by specialized cells called osteoclasts and new bone tissue is formed by osteoblasts. This dynamic process, called osteogenesis, helps maintain bone strength, repair micro-damage, and adapt to changes in mechanical stress. By understanding the processes of bone development, growth, and maintenance, individuals can take proactive steps to support optimal bone health throughout life and reduce the risk of osteoporosis and fractures. Regular exercise, a balanced diet, and lifestyle modifications play key roles in promoting strong and healthy bones.monitoring changes that may be occurring in the musculoskeletal system as we age; individuals can promote optimal bone health, reduce the risk of fractures, and maintain mobility and independence throughout the lifespan.

3

The Basics of Bone Health

The basics of bone health encompass understanding the anatomy of bones, bone development, and strategies to maintain optimal bone density and strength. Bones are living tissues composed of collagen, calcium phosphate and calcium carbonate, and a dozen other minerals. They are not stiff, nor solid, but living, bending material that is both strong and flexible and able to withstand incredible amounts of stress or loading. In fact, loading or weight bearing actually stimulates bone growth as the bones respond to the stress by building more density and strength. Bones consist of a harder outer layer called cortical bone and a spongy and honeycombed interior called trabecular bone. It is said that the entire skeleton regenerates itself every 7-10 years.

Bones begin to grow in the womb and can be seen on ultrasound as early as 9 weeks with the mandible, scapula, clavicle and long bones ossifying by 12-16 weeks. The spine can be seen clearly in routine 20 week ultrasounds. Childhood and adolescence are critical periods for bone growth and development. During these stages, bones undergo rapid growth and increase in length, width, and density. Bone growth occurs primarily at the growth plates, which are areas of cartilage located near the ends of long bones. Hormones, particularly growth hormone and sex hormones (estrogen and testosterone), play key roles in regulating bone growth and development during puberty. Adequate nutrition, including sufficient intake of calcium, vitamin D, protein, and other essential nutrients, is crucial for supporting optimal bone growth and mineralization during childhood and adolescence

During this period, bones grow and increase in size through a process called bone remodeling, which involves the removal of old bone tissue by specialized cells called osteoclasts and the formation of new bone tissue by osteoblasts. This process is happening constantly as the cells in the bones turnover and rebuild; however as individuals age and particularly as hormone levels change during the aging process, there can be an imbalance in the process that allows more bone to be removed than what is rebuilt. Peak bone mass occurs in early adulthood by age 30, with most musculoskeletal development occurring by age 18 or 20. Women reach their peak sooner than men. Regular weight bearing exercise and activity is usually enough to maintain bone density until about age 40, when most begin to lose some bone density, around 1% per year on average.

Bone Density and Strength

Throughout the book, we refer to bone density and strength, character-istics intimately connected to bone health. Bone density is the amount of mineral content in the bone tissue and is a key factor in determining bone strength. Bone mineral density or BMD measures the amount of minerals in the bone, primarily calcium and phosphorus, because the more minerals in the bones, the denser and stronger the bones are and stronger bones are less likely to fracture. Optimal bone density and strength are essential in delivering those foundational benefits like supporting the body's weight, absorbing shock, and resisting fractures.

Bone density is closely related to overall strength and physical function. Here's how:

- **Structural Support:** Bones provide structural support for the body, allowing us to stand, move, and perform daily activities. Bone density refers to the amount of mineral content in bone tissue, and denser bones are stronger and better able to withstand mechanical stress and load-bearing activities.
- **Resistance to Fractures:** Higher bone density is associated with greater bone strength and resilience, reducing the risk of fractures, particularly fragility fractures that occur with minimal trauma or force. Individuals with low bone density are more susceptible to fractures, which can lead to pain, disability, and limitations in mobility and function.
- **Muscle Attachment:** Bones serve as attachment sites for muscles, tendons, and ligaments, facilitating movement and providing leverage for muscle action. Stronger bones provide a more stable foundation for muscle attachment, enabling efficient muscle function and optimal physical performance.
- **Balance and Stability:** Bone density influences balance and stability, which are essential for maintaining posture, preventing falls, and avoiding injuries. Strong bones provide better support and stability, reducing the risk of falls and improving overall balance and coordination.
- **Joint Health:** Strong bones help maintain joint integrity and function by providing support and protection for the surrounding joint structures. Higher bone density can reduce the risk of joint degeneration and osteoarthritis, which can impair mobility and quality of life.

- **Overall Strength and Function:** Strong bones contribute to overall physical strength and functional capacity, allowing individuals to engage in activities of daily living, participate in sports and recreational activities, and maintain independence and quality of life.

In summary, bone density is a critical determinant of bone strength and overall musculoskeletal health. Maintaining optimal bone density through proper nutrition, weight-bearing exercise, and lifestyle modifications is essential for promoting bone strength, preventing fractures, and preserving physical function and mobility throughout life.

Factors that Influence Bone Density

There are many factors that influence bone density and strength include genetics, nutrition, physical activity, hormonal balance, and lifestyle habits. Each of these topics could fill and entire chapter if not an entire book, but we will give a high level overview.

While genetics play an important role, bone mineral density and osteoporosis is impacted by the influence of several genes, not just one mutation of a single gene. Sometimes, just being aware of your family history is enough to help understand that part of your risk. Studies show that genetic factors are important in the development of bone density itself, as well as other inherited bio markers such as body mass index and the onset of menstruation and menopause. There may also be genetic factors that contribute to the structure and geometry of the bones themselves. What we do know is that while genetics plays a role, it is not the only important factor to consider. There are many other factors to consider, factors over which we have more control and opportunity to improve our risk factors.

Nutrition is everyone's starting point in building and maintaining healthy bones and it starts in childhood. Poor nutrition in childhood, particularly diets low in calcium and vitamin D, can sabotage a child's ability to grow to typical peak bone mass. Eating disorders during childhood or teen years can also cause malnutrition, negatively affecting their peak bone mass at a crucial time in a child's development. Bone loss due to anorexia nervosa can be seen in as little as 6 months and deficits can remain even after recovery. It has been suggested that achieving peak bone mass during these formative years can delay the onset of age related osteoporosis by as much as 13 years, further reducing the risk of fracture during the senior years when a fracture is most dangerous. Nutrition is not just for the young and plays a crucial role in maintaining a healthy foundation at all stages of life. During childhood and adolescence, however, much more bone is added to the skeleton than is removed, growing the bones and building density that can be impactful decades later. A separate section is included on nutrition with specifics on foods that support bone health.

Calcium and vitamin D are essential nutrients for bone health throughout life. Calcium is required for bone mineralization and vitamin D facilitates calcium absorption and utilization. There are, however, other essentials for good bone health and these include vitamin k2, magnesium, phosphorus and good quality protein. Other minerals with a key role to play include zinc which is required for bone mineralization and boron which aids the body in utilizing other minerals. Copper and iron play a role as do vitamins A, C, and all the B vitamins. It becomes easy to understand why overall good nutrition is so important, not just calcium intake. Another thing to consider is in recent years calcium supplementation has come under fire for causing kidney stones and colon polyps. Yet another study has linked calcium supplementation to calcium buildup in the arteries contributing to heart attacks and heart disease. The good news is that calcium is relatively easy to get in the diet, with planning and awareness of what foods are rich and easy to consume daily.

Physical activity is also an important part of maintaining or improving bone health. Physical activity in childhood improves bone mineralization and structure and lays a foundation of good skeletal health that may prevent osteoporosis in later life. Weight-bearing exercises, such as hiking, walking, running, dancing, and strength training, stimulate bone remodeling and help maintain bone density and strength at any age. Regular physical activity also improves balance, coordination, and muscle strength, reducing the risk of falls and fractures. New fitness technologies like OsteoStrong offer an easy and efficient solution to improving strength and many users have confirmed bone density improvements confirmed through x-ray scans called DEXA scans.

Lifestyle modifications are a third way to improve outcomes with regard to long-term bone health. Avoiding smoking and excessive alcohol consumption is important as these habits can negatively impact bone density and increase fracture risk. Smoking reduces blood supply to the bones and the nicotine slows production of osteoblasts, the bone building cells. Smoking also inhibits the body's ability to absorb calcium, which is necessary for many cellular functions in the body in addition to providing the foundation of strong bones. Additionally smokers take longer to heal from fractures. Smoking also causes inflammation throughout the body which contributes to conditions like osteoporosis among others. Alcohol is known to increase cortisol, also called as the stress hormone, which decreases osteoblast production or bone building activity and increases osteoclast activity which contributes to further breakdown of bone. Alcohol abuse is also known to increase parathyroid hormone, an excess of which pulls calcium from the bones.

Finally, being aware of hormonal changes in the body is an action that can help you stay proactive in your bone health journey. Hormones such as estrogen, testosterone, growth hormone, and thyroid hormones regulate bone metabolism and influence bone density. Thyroid hormones are essential for bone remodeling and low or high levels can impact bone health in both children and adults. Estrogen is a great bone protector and stimulates osteoblast production throughout life. The sharp decline in estrogen during menopause is responsible for delivering many a shocking DEXA score, often to active women who thought they were in "good health". This was my story, despite my active sports related fractures, I felt I was fit and had been eating an organic, Mediterranean diet for years. I felt great, without aches or pain. But menopause is full of surprises, but in this book we will stay focused on bone health

The Impact of Menopause

Menopause can have a significant impact on bone health due to the hormonal changes that occur during this transition. Statistically in the United States, one out of two women over 50 will break a bone due to low bone density. Menopause impacts every woman, so we will include some specific here on how menopause affects the bones:

- **Estrogen Decline:** During menopause, a woman's ovaries gradually produce less estrogen, leading to a decline in circulating estrogen levels. Estrogen plays a crucial role in maintaining bone density by inhibiting bone breakdown and promoting bone formation. The decrease in estrogen levels during menopause can accelerate bone loss, particularly in trabecular bone (spongy bone tissue), which is more responsive to hormonal changes.
- **Accelerated Bone Loss:** In the first few years after menopause, women may experience accelerated bone loss, with bone density

declining at a faster rate than before menopause. This phase of rapid bone loss is known as postmenopausal osteoporosis and can increase the risk of fractures, especially in weight-bearing bones such as the spine, hips, and wrists.

- **Increased Fracture Risk:** The decline in bone density and strength during menopause increases the risk of fractures, particularly fragility fractures (fractures that occur with minimal trauma or force). Common sites for fractures in postmenopausal women include the vertebrae (spine), hip, and wrist.
- **Bone Remodeling Imbalance:** Estrogen deficiency alters the balance between bone resorption (breakdown) and bone formation, leading to increased bone turnover and a net loss of bone tissue. This imbalance in bone remodeling contributes to bone fragility and susceptibility to fractures.
- **Changes in Bone Structure:** Estrogen deficiency during menopause can also affect bone structure, leading to alterations in bone architecture and quality. Trabecular bone becomes more porous and less dense, while cortical bone (dense outer layer) may become thinner and more susceptible to fractures.
- **Other Factors:** In addition to estrogen decline, other factors associated with menopause, such as age-related muscle loss (sarcopenia), changes in body composition, and lifestyle factors (e.g., decreased physical activity, smoking, inadequate nutrition), can further exacerbate bone loss and increase fracture risk.

Overall, menopause represents a critical period of vulnerability for bone health in women, highlighting the importance of proactive measures to preserve bone density and reduce fracture risk. Lifestyle modifications, including weight-bearing exercise, adequate calcium and vitamin D intake, and avoidance of smoking and excessive alcohol consumption, are essential for maintaining bone health during and after menopause.

Another important part of managing bone health as we age is monitoring changes that may be occurring in the aging body. Osteoporosis is called the silent disease because it is often completely painless and symptom free until a fracture occurs. Knowing your risk factors, completing regular check-ups, and securing bone density tests can help monitor bone health and identify any abnormalities or deficiencies early on. DEXA, or dual-energy X-ray absorptiometry is a medical imaging text which has been the primary tool used to diagnose osteoporosis since 1988. While guidelines for when to receive a DEXA scan vary, many women are not covered by insurance until age 65. However, if you know your risk factors, you can ask your doctor to write a prescription for a DEXA scan based on those risk factors; say a family history of osteoporosis, a teenage eating disorder, and a fracture.

As with all medical interactions, advocate for yourself with your primary care physician if you have concerns about your bone density. If they are not responsive to your concerns, find another doctor. If that is not an option for you, find an outlet that offers ultrasound heel scans, generally offered for free at health fairs and corporate wellness events. While not a tool for diagnosis, it is a safe way to get feedback on your bone density in one area of the body and the machine produces a report that can be shared with your doctor

Additionally, healthcare providers may recommend bone density testing and, if necessary, pharmacological interventions to prevent or treat osteoporosis in postmenopausal women at high risk of fractures. A note of caution here however, traditional therapies for treating osteoporosis are often limited to pharmaceutical interventions and may not be the first solution individuals may want to try when faced with a diagnosis of osteoporosis and evaluating the potential of benefits over the potential side-effects. That is one of the primary reasons for awareness and practices that support bone health from an early age as well as understanding the practices that support bone health in a holistic and natural way throughout a lifetime, practices without negative side effects and many long-term benefits.

By incorporating these basic principles of bone health into daily life, bone health supporting nutrition, weight bearing exercise, a healthy lifestyle free of smoking and alcohol abuse as well as monitoring changes that may be occurring in the musculoskeletal system as we age; individuals can promote optimal bone health, reduce the risk of fractures, and maintain mobility and independence throughout the lifespan.

Bone Development and Growth

To recap, an individual's peak bone mass, or the maximum amount of bone tissue a person can attain, is a good determinant of future bone health issues. Achieving optimal peak bone mass during adolescence and young adulthood is important for reducing the risk of osteoporosis and fractures later in life. Throughout life, bones undergo a continuous process of remodeling, where old bone tissue is resorbed by specialized cells called osteoclasts and new bone tissue is formed by osteoblasts. This dynamic process, called osteogenesis, helps maintain bone strength, repair micro-damage, and adapt to changes in mechanical stress. By understanding the processes of bone development, growth, and maintenance, individuals can take proactive steps to support optimal bone health throughout life and reduce the risk of osteoporosis and fractures. Regular exercise, a balanced diet, and lifestyle modifications play key roles in promoting strong and healthy bones.

4

Understanding Fractures

Fractures are a great burden on the medical system. Over $59 billion per year is spent by private insurance, medicare and medicaid in medical services, hospital stays and equipment related to falls and fractures. A person who endures a fracture will have 4 times the medical costs in a year than one without a fracture incidence. And these statistics do not include the personal costs which might include additional care in the home, transportation if unable to drive, lost wages, and the more long term issues of isolation and loneliness as people withdraw from activities they cannot do or are afraid to do. Several factors can increase an individual's risk of fractures. Those at higher risk typically include:

- **Age**: Older adults, especially those over 65, are at increased risk due to age-related changes in bone density, muscle strength, and balance, as well as a higher likelihood of chronic health conditions and medication use.
- **Gender**: Women are more prone to fractures, particularly after menopause, due to the rapid decline in estrogen levels, which accelerates bone loss and increases the risk of osteoporosis.

- **Bone Health**: Individuals with low bone density or osteoporosis are at greater risk of fractures, as their bones are weaker and more prone to breakage.
- **Medical Conditions**: Certain medical conditions, such as osteoporosis, osteogenesis imperfecta, rheumatoid arthritis, and cancer, can weaken bones and increase fracture risk.
- **Medication Use:** Some medications, including corticosteroids, anticoagulants, and certain antidepressants, can weaken bones or increase the risk of falls, thereby predisposing individuals to fractures.
- **Nutritional Deficiencies**: Inadequate intake of calcium, vitamin D, and other essential nutrients necessary for bone health can increase fracture risk.
- **Family History**: A family history of osteoporosis or fractures may indicate a genetic predisposition to bone-related issues and increase an individual's fracture risk.
- **Lifestyle Factors:** Certain lifestyle habits, such as smoking, excessive alcohol consumption, sedentary behavior, and poor nutrition, can negatively impact bone health and increase fracture risk.
- **Environmental Hazards**: Occupational hazards, recreational activities, and environmental factors in the home or community settings can increase the likelihood of falls and fractures.
- **Previous Fractures**: Individuals who have previously experienced fractures may be at higher risk of subsequent fractures due to compromised bone integrity and altered biomechanics.
- **Cognitive Impairment:** Conditions such as dementia or Alzheimer's disease can impair judgment, coordination, and balance, increasing the risk of falls and fractures.
- **Mobility Impairments**: Conditions that affect mobility, such as Parkinson's disease, stroke, or lower limb disabilities, can increase the risk of falls and fractures.

Identifying and addressing these risk factors is crucial for implementing preventive measures and interventions aimed at reducing fracture risk and promoting bone health across the lifespan. By adopting a proactive approach to bone health, individuals can minimize their risk of fractures and maintain a high quality of life

In order to better understand the risk of fracture, a simple overview of the types and causes of fractures are detailed here. If a reader unfortunately suffers a fracture, they will have some familiarity with the terms they will no doubt hear during their diagnosis.

Types of Fractures: Fractures can vary in severity and presentation. Common types include:

- **Closed Fracture:** The bone breaks but does not penetrate the skin.
- **Open Fracture:** Also known as a compound fracture, where the broken bone pierces through the skin.
- **Stress Fracture:** A hairline crack in the bone caused by repetitive stress or overuse.
- **Comminuted Fracture:** The bone shatters into multiple pieces.
- **Compression Fracture:** The bone collapses or is crushed, often seen in vertebrae due to osteoporosis.
- **Avulsion Fracture:** A fragment of bone is pulled away by a tendon or ligament.

Causes of Fractures: Fractures can occur due to various factors, including:

- **Trauma:** Falls, accidents, sports injuries, or direct blows to the bone.
- **Overuse:** Repetitive stress or strain on the bone, commonly seen in athletes or individuals engaged in high-impact activities.

- **Medical Conditions:** Conditions like osteoporosis, osteogenesis imperfecta, or bone cancer can weaken bones and increase fracture risk.
- **Medications:** Some medications can also cause low bone density and increase fracture risk such as proton pump inhibitors used as common heartburn drugs, or aromatase inhibitors used in breast cancer treatments. Your doctor should make you aware of bone loss as side effect of any medications as this can be a life threatening complication.
- **Age:** Older adults are more prone to fractures due to age-related changes in bone density and strength.
- **Nutritional Deficiencies:** Inadequate intake of calcium, vitamin D, and other essential nutrients can weaken bones and predispose individuals to fractures.

Symptoms: Signs of a fracture may include:

- Pain, swelling, and tenderness at the site of the injury.
- Bruising or discoloration.
- Deformity or abnormal alignment of the affected limb.
- Inability to bear weight or move the injured area.

Diagnosis: Fractures are typically diagnosed through a combination of physical examination, imaging tests (X-rays, CT scans, MRI), and medical history assessment.

Treatment: Treatment for fractures depends on the type and severity of the injury but may include:

- Immobilization with a cast, brace, or splint.
- Reduction, which involves realigning the broken bone fragments.

- Surgery to stabilize the fracture with pins, plates, screws, or rods.
- Rehabilitation exercises to restore strength, flexibility, and function.

Understanding the different types, causes, symptoms, diagnosis, and treatment of fractures is essential for asking questions during treatment and effectively managing injuries and minimizing their impact on overall health and well-being. Early recognition and prompt treatment can facilitate healing and reduce the risk of long-term complications associated with fractures.

Fractures are a challenge no matter what age they occur; however fractures in the elderly are both a significant risk to the patient's overall quality of life and potentially even a cause of mortality. According to the National Institute of Health falls are considered a leading cause of injury and death among individuals 65 and older. A fear of falling also contributes to individuals withdrawing from activities that are perceived as more likely to present fall risks. These activities are often activities that involve positive social aspects and personal satisfaction, resulting in a reduction in quality of life for that person. While the causes of falls in the elderly reflect the same causes we see across the population, the impact, no pun intended, can be far more significant for seniors than other segments of the population.

Causes of Fractures Among the Elderly:

Every aging person would likely agree that maintaining their indepen-dence and high quality of life is a top priority. However a major threat to this desire is the loss of musculoskeletal strength and muscle mass which causes a loss of mobility and function. For many, this is a foregone conclusion and one that is is direct conflict with how most individuals want to age.

Osteoporosis is a common condition characterized by low bone density and weakened bones, making bones more susceptible to fractures, particularly in the hip, spine, and wrist. As people age, bone density naturally decreases, increasing the risk of osteoporosis and associated fractures. Both women and men are prone to osteoporosis as they age. Women, due to menopause see more significant loss of BMD earlier than men; however men also experience age-related BMD decline. The all too familiar sloping shoulders and rounded back are common among both men and women as they lose bone and muscle strength.

Falls are a leading cause of fractures among the elderly population. Factors contributing to falls include muscle weakness, blood pressure regulation, impaired balance and coordination, vision or hearing problems, medication side effects, environmental hazards such as slippery floors or poor lighting.

Certain medical conditions prevalent among older adults, such as osteoarthritis, rheumatoid arthritis, and Parkinson's disease, can increase the risk of fractures due to weakened bones, joint instability, or impaired mobility. Dementia can also contribute to an increased fall risk in seniors.

Inadequate intake of essential nutrients, particularly calcium and vitamin D, can contribute to bone loss and increase fracture risk among the elderly. Poor nutrition, malabsorption syndromes, and dietary restrictions may further exacerbate this risk. Many seniors are also challenged to eat enough protein as they age which is essential to building and maintaining bone and muscle mass and strength.

Certain medications commonly prescribed to older adults, such as corticosteroids, anticoagulants, and sedatives, can weaken bones, increase the risk of falls, or impair balance and coordination, thereby predisposing individuals to fractures. A change in medication or dose of medication can also cause changes in balance. Be certain to include questions about the impact to bone health when speaking to health care providers.

Sedentary lifestyles and decreased physical activity levels, whether due to aging, chronic illness, or mobility limitations, can lead to muscle weakness, decreased bone density, and impaired balance, all of which contribute to an increased risk of fractures. Sadly, some diagnosis like that of osteoporosis creates fear of falling and fracturing which dissuades individuals from movement and physical activities which are essential to maintaining strength and mobility.

Environmental factors in the home or community settings, such as uneven surfaces, clutter, inadequate lighting, and lack of handrails or grab bars, can pose hazards and increase the likelihood of falls and fractures among the elderly. Unfortunately for many folks as they age, it becomes more difficult to keep up with housework and yard work, potentially creating situations where the environment deteriorates with more clutter and disarray.

Chronic health conditions prevalent in older adults, such as diabetes, cardiovascular disease, and stroke, may indirectly contribute to fractures by affecting mobility, cognitive function, or overall health status.

Understanding these common causes of fractures among the elderly is essential for implementing preventive measures and interventions aimed at reducing fracture risk, promoting bone health, and enhancing overall well-being in this vulnerable population. By addressing modifiable risk factors and implementing strategies to improve bone strength, mobility, and safety, we can help mitigate the impact of fractures and improve the quality of life for older adults.

35

_5_

Fall-proofing the Home Environment

A key preventative measure we can take to prevent broken bones is to fall-proof the home. Whether you are considering your own home or perhaps the home of someone for whom you are a care giver, it is essential to use a critical eye to evaluate and improve the home environment from a fracture risk perspective. This is, for the most part, an easy and inexpensive measure; although some homes might benefit from more expensive remodeling type projects, like a first floor bathroom addition for example, this chapter will concentrate on things _everyone_ can do to make the home a safer environment. This of course is important throughout a lifetime, it is especially important during the senior years when fractures can have life changing impacts reducing independence and quality of life, often in a very brief period of time.

One dangerous condition in a home environment that can cause falls is clutter. Whether one is young or not young, clutter creates hazards that can impede free movement through the home and create opportunities for trips and falls. Clutter can be as simple as shoes slipped off and discarded in an arrival and departure zone or more severe clutter such as that which can be seen in age-related hoarding, which affects three times the adults over 55 than it does those 34-44 years of age. In younger families, it may be toys and school related items like backpacks and instrument cases that may be left in traffic locations that can add fall risk to quickly moving youngsters and their parents. Whatever the out of place items are, it is important to make a practice of putting items away, keeping things tidy, out of walking paths and off of stairs.

Stairways for obvious reasons are an area of special concern. Handrails are crucial, and should on both sides of the stairs if possible. Making a practice of using the railings, especially when carrying something, adds a safety measure that can quickly steady a person and keep them from a tumble that could have dire results. Stairs should be well lit and have light switches at the top and bottom. Motion activated lights can offer an easy solution to turning lights off and on easily, particularly overnight. Outside staircases should have non-slip surfaces as well.

Other preventative measure to fall-proof a home include removing slippery throw rugs or using no-slip strips to keep them firmly in place. All carpets should be firmly attached to the floor and without wrinkles and other imperfections rising up the trip up a passerby. Wet floors can also be treacherous and caution should be taken around freshly washed floors. Consider purchasing a plastic floor sign for a an easily recognized reminder of a wet floor. For the same reasons, spills should be cleaned immediately.

Bathrooms have many hard surfaces which can become quite slippery when wet. Firmly mounted grab bars near toilets and inside and outside of showers and bathtubs offer secure assistance when needed, bathmats should be non-skid and should be used in areas that will likely get wet. A night light is also highly recommended in the bathroom, one that turns on and off automatically in the dark is preferred.Bedrooms also benefit from night lights and light switches should be easily reached. Keeping a small flashlight near the bed can be helpful, especially if there is a power outage. Access to a phone is also recommended for the bedside, primarily for older individuals.

The kitchen has some special recommendations for easier and safer functionality: keep pots, pans and utensils in easy to reach storage. This may involve reworking the way items are stored in the cupboards and cabinets but can definitely make life easier and safer. Heavy items like pots and pans are often stored in low cabinets which may require more effort for anyone with strength or fragility issues. Another thing to consider for enhanced safety in the kitchen, especially for anyone recovering from an injury or for someone with balance issues is to prepare food while seated. While this may be a foreign concept for some, it will immediately add stability to the process when needed. This can also prevent fatigue. Good kitchen practices for fall-proofing also include cleaning spills that make it to the floor immediately, and always using a step stool with a handle or using a grabbing -device for hard to reach items.

Areas of transition, or places that allow inside and outside access from in or around the home deserve a special review. Steps should be in good condition and free of any broken elements, hand railings should be in place even if it is just 3 steps. Lighting should be available and utilized in advance for after dark returns and if balance is an issue, consider a grab bar in the doorway area between inside and outside of the home, which can assist with balance issues and provide mobility assistance as needed.

In any area of the home, keep electrical cords out of the way, along a wall if possible. Arrange furniture so that there is a clear path and easy flow around low items like coffee tables. Chairs should be at a height that is easy to get in and out of without struggle or assistance. Never stand on a chair to reach a high spot and always use a step stool with a hand rail. For extra protection, have someone stand near you while on the step stool especially if balance is an issue.

Pets can be our best friends but are also often under foot and are a very reliable trip-hazard. Most pet owners will have a story or two of nearly falling over or due to the actions of their pets. Be aware of your pet's location whenever moving or walking. Everyone, but especially seniors, should be cautious when walking large powerful dogs and individuals with any mobility or balance issues should consider the possibility of losing control of their animal and the potential ramifications of that. There are many dog walking services and should be considered as an option when fall risk is great. Additionally, fencing a portion of the yard can help a senior dog owner keep a pet in the home when mobility is an issue.

In conclusion, a fall can be a life altering occasion and action should be employed to prevent falls, especially in the home and especially for vulnerable populations like small children and the elderly or infirm.

A fall-proofing recap for easy reference:

- Reduce clutter.
- Make certain stairways are well lit and have firmly attached handrails.
- Exterior stairs should have non-slip surfaces.
- Keep electrical cords against walls and away from traffic areas..
- Use porch lights, nightlights and motion lights.
- Use Grab bars in bathrooms and transition areas.

- Clean up spills and don't walk on wet surfaces.
- Consider rearranging the kitchen for easy access of the most often used items.
- Consider sitting while preparing food.
- Furniture should be placed for ease of movement and hazard free flow..
- Chairs should be sturdy and at a comfortable height for getting up and down.
- Use a step ladder with a handrail and a spotter.
- Be aware of pets.

6

Supporting Bone Health with Diet and Nutrition

few thoughts on diet and nutrition: entire books have been written on just this subject and I would highly recommend any of Dr. Mark Hyman's books or Lara Pizzorno's *Healthy Bones Healthy You!* These authors can provide great overall information as well as in depth and detailed nutritional studies and recommendations. My favorite and go-to cookbook is *The Healthy Bones Nutrition Plan and Cookbook.* I find the recipes tasty and appealing to everyone at the table and allow me to be provide bone healthy meals easily.

This book would not be complete, even as a quick guide to bone health without a section on diet and eating for bone health. I will preface the section by admitting this is just scratching the surface on the subject. But I will try to provide a good place to start. Preventing fractures through nutrition and diet is crucial for maintaining optimal bone health and strength. Most will agree, this is where to start any bone health journey. Here are some key dietary factors to consider:

Calcium is the primary mineral responsible for building and maintaining bone density. Most adults need 1000-1200 milligrams per day. The definition of a 'good source' of calcium means there is at least 10% or more of the daily recommended amount. Adequate calcium intake is essential for supporting bone health and reducing the risk of fractures. Good food sources of calcium include dairy products (plain or greek yogurt, hard cheeses, cottage and ricotta cheese, kefir), leafy green vegetables (cooked kale, broccoli, bok choy, turnip or collard greens), tofu, canned seafood (salmon or sardines), oranges, mineral water, almonds, figs, white beans, and fortified foods (orange juice, cereals).

Vitamin D is necessary for calcium absorption and utilization in the body. Without sufficient vitamin D, calcium cannot be effectively absorbed, leading to weakened bones and increased fracture risk. One's needs increase with age with children needing around 600 daily IU and adults 800-1000 IU. Sunlight exposure, fatty fish (e.g., salmon, mackerel), and egg yolks are sources of vitamin D. In some cases, supplementation may be necessary, especially for individuals with limited sun exposure or vitamin D deficiency. If you live in a northern climate, supplementation is recommended October-May.

Protein is essential for bone health, as it provides the building blocks necessary for bone formation and repair. Including adequate protein in the diet supports bone strength and reduces the risk of fractures. Protein recommendations are typically around 60 grams of protein per day for a 150 pound woman and 65 grams for a 180 pound man. Seniors however may require higher amounts due to numerous reasons from inflammation to medication to active lifestyle, some sources say as much as 30% more. Good sources of protein include lean meats, poultry, fish, eggs, dairy products, legumes, nuts, and seeds. Single sources with large contributions include salmon 3 oz = 22 g, greek yogurt 7 oz = 20 g, chicken 4 oz = 24 g, lentils 1 c = 18 g, 1 cottage cheese 1 c = 25 g, 1 egg = 6 g, bottle of mineral water = 10–12 g.

Magnesium plays a role in bone metabolism and is involved in the regulation of calcium levels in the body. Daily recommendations are around 300 mg. However, magnesium is one supplement that can cause problems at higher doses so please be cautious and seek the advice of a medical professional. Consuming magnesium-rich foods, such as nuts, seeds, whole grains, leafy green vegetables, and legumes, and even dark chocolate (50-90% cocoa solids), support bone health and reduce fracture risk.

Vitamin K2 is involved in bone mineralization and helps maintain bone density. Of particular interest to folks with low bone density is vitamin K2-7 or menaquinone-7 or MK-7. This is a special type of vitamin K with higher bioavailability that has benefits for osteoporosis as well as cardiovascular and dementia diseases. Fermented foods such as natto are good sources of vitamin K2 as are meats, cheeses and eggs. A more powerful option to choose however, are pasture raised animal products as they deliver the more bioavailable MK-7. Look for grass fed and grass finished options for the highest quality.

Phosphorus, next to calcium,is most prevalent mineral in the body and roughly 80% of it is found in our bones and teeth. Phosphorus is another mineral that contributes to bone structure and strength and in fact signs of a phosphorous deficiency include bone pain. In children, a deficiency of phosphorus will contribute to weak bones and teeth. Foods rich in phosphorus include dairy products, meat, poultry, fish, nuts, seeds, and whole grains.

Vitamin C is important for collagen synthesis, which is essential for bone formation and structure.Collagen provides the framework upon which minerals are deposited during bone mineralization. Citrus fruits, berries, kiwi, bell peppers, broccoli, and tomatoes are good sources of vitamin C.

Vitamin A is involved in bone remodeling and the maintenance of bone density. Excessive intake of vitamin A from supplements can have negative effects on bone health, but adequate intake from dietary sources is beneficial. Good dietary sources of vitamin A include liver, fish oil, eggs, dairy products, and orange and yellow fruits and vegetables (such as carrots, sweet potatoes, and cantaloupe.

Zinc plays a role in bone formation and mineralization and is involved in the synthesis of collagen and bone proteins. Zinc deficiency can impair bone growth and development and increase the risk of fractures. Dietary sources of zinc include meat, poultry, fish, shellfish, nuts, seeds, whole grains, and legumes.

Boron is a trace mineral that may help support bone health by influencing calcium and magnesium metabolism and promoting bone mineralization. Research suggests that boron supplementation may improve bone density and reduce the risk of osteoporosis. Dietary sources of boron include fruits (such as apples, grapes, and avocados), nuts, legumes, and whole grains.

Limiting Sodium and Caffeine are two more easy opportunities for improving the diet and supporting bone health. High sodium intake can increase calcium excretion in the urine, leading to decreased calcium availability for bone health. Similarly, excessive caffeine consumption may interfere with calcium absorption. Moderating intake of salty foods and caffeinated beverages can help preserve bone density.

A Balanced Diet is one of the best ways to pursue a strong bones lifestyle. Consuming a balanced diet rich in fruits, vegetables, whole grains, lean proteins, and healthy fats provides essential nutrients for overall health, including bone health. Avoiding restrictive diets and ensuring adequate calorie intake is important for maintaining optimal bone density and strength. By prioritizing nutrient-rich foods and adopting a balanced diet, individuals can support bone health, reduce fracture risk, and maintain overall well-being. It's also important to consult with a healthcare provider or registered dietitian for personalized nutrition recommendations based on individual health status and dietary needs.

Dietary Concerns of Aging

As individuals age, there are certain dietary risks that can negatively impact bone health and increase the risk of fractures. Becoming aware of these challenges is the first step in finding appropriate solutions. Some of these dietary risks include:

Reduced Nutrient Absorption: Aging is associated with changes in digestion and nutrient absorption, which can affect the body's ability to utilize essential nutrients for bone health, such as calcium, vitamin D, and vitamin K.

Decreased Appetite: Older adults may experience a decreased appetite due to factors such as changes in taste perception, medications, dental issues, or chronic health conditions. This may result in inadequate nutrient intake, including calcium and protein, which are important for bone health.

Limited Sun Exposure: Vitamin D synthesis in the skin decreases with age, and older adults may spend less time outdoors, further reducing their exposure to sunlight, which is necessary for vitamin D production. This can lead to vitamin D deficiency, impairing calcium absorption and negatively impacting bone health.

Medication Interactions: Older adults are more likely to be taking multiple medications, some of which may affect bone health. For example, certain medications, such as corticosteroids, anticonvulsants, proton pump inhibitors, and diuretics, can interfere with calcium absorption or increase the risk of bone loss.

Chronic Health Conditions: Aging is often accompanied by the development of chronic health conditions, such as osteoporosis, osteoarthritis, kidney disease, or gastrointestinal disorders, which can impact nutrient absorption, metabolism, or utilization, affecting bone health.

Dental Issues: Poor dental health or tooth loss can make it difficult for older adults to chew and digest nutrient-rich foods, leading to dietary deficiencies that may affect bone health.

Altered Taste and Smell: Changes in taste and smell perception with age may affect food preferences and intake, potentially leading to a less varied diet and reduced consumption of nutrient-dense foods important for bone health.

Inadequate Hydration: Dehydration is common among older adults and can affect calcium balance and bone density. Maintaining adequate hydration is important for overall health, including bone health.

Socioeconomic Factors: Socioeconomic factors, such as limited access to nutritious foods, financial constraints, or living in food-insecure environments, may contribute to poor dietary choices and nutritional deficiencies that impact bone health.

Addressing these dietary risks through strategies such as optimizing nutrient intake, addressing medication interactions, promoting oral health, encouraging physical activity, and addressing socioeconomic barriers can help support bone health and reduce the risk of fractures as individuals age. Regular monitoring of bone health and consultation with healthcare providers or registered dietitians can also help identify and address specific dietary needs and risks in older adults.

7

Physical Activity and Bone Density

P hysical activity plays a crucial role in promoting bone health and reducing the risk of fractures. Bone strength and development starts as as a toddler, wobbling and falling down, continuing through childhood as we run and jump, and still is building to peak bone density as individuals enter their teenage years with organized sports commitments and the emergence of physical talents, right into adulthood where physical activity starts to play a supporting role, more so than the main attraction. Here's how physical activity contributes to bone health and fracture prevention throughout your lifetime:

Weight-Bearing Exercise: Weight-bearing activities, which require the body to work against gravity, stimulate bone remodeling and help maintain bone density and strength. Examples of weight-bearing exercises include walking, jogging, dancing, stair climbing, hiking, and strength training with weights or resistance bands.

Impact and High-Intensity Exercise: Activities that involve impact and high-intensity movements, such as running, jumping, and plyometrics, exert mechanical stress on bones, promoting bone formation and mineralization.These activities are particularly effective at stimulating bone growth and strengthening bones in children, adolescents, and young adults.

Resistance Training: Resistance training, also known as strength training or weightlifting, involves using external resistance (such as free weights, weight machines, or resistance bands) to build muscle strength and endurance. Resistance training not only strengthens muscles but also places stress on bones, leading to improvements in bone density and strength.

Balance and Coordination Exercises: Balance and coordination exercises, such as yoga, Tai chi, and Pilates, improve proprioception (awareness of body position) and neuromuscular control, reducing the risk of falls and fractures.These activities also help maintain mobility, stability, and functional independence, which are important for preventing fall-related injuries.

Functional Movement Patterns: Incorporating functional movement patterns into exercise routines helps improve joint mobility, flexibility, and range of motion, reducing the risk of musculoskeletal injuries. Functional exercises mimic activities of daily living and promote efficient movement mechanics, which can help prevent falls and fractures.

Moderate Physical Activity: Engaging in regular moderate-intensity physical activity, such as brisk walking, cycling, swimming, or gardening, provides overall health benefits and supports bone health. While moderate-intensity activities may not exert as much mechanical stress on bones as high-impact or weight-bearing exercises, they still contribute to maintaining mobility, cardiovascular health, and overall well-being.

Lifestyle Factors: In addition to structured exercise, adopting a physically active lifestyle that includes regular movement throughout the day (such as taking the stairs, standing up frequently, or participating in recreational activities) can help maintain bone health and reduce the risk of fractures.

By incorporating a variety of weight-bearing, impact, resistance, balance, and functional exercises into one's routine, individuals can promote optimal bone health, reduce the risk of fractures, and maintain mobility and independence throughout life. It's important to consult with a healthcare provider or qualified fitness professional to develop a safe and effective exercise program tailored to individual needs, preferences, and health goals.

Weight bearing Exercise and Bone Health

The best weight-bearing exercises for bone health are those that require you to work against gravity while standing upright, stimulating bone remodeling and helping to maintain bone density and strength. Here are some of the most effective weight-bearing exercises for bone health:

- **Walking:** Walking is a simple and accessible weight-bearing exercise that can be done almost anywhere. It is low-impact and suitable for people of all ages and fitness levels. Aim for brisk walking for at least 30 minutes most days of the week to reap the bone-strengthening benefits.
- **Jogging/Running:** Jogging or running provides a higher impact stimulus to the bones compared to walking, making it more effective for improving bone density. However, it may not be suitable for everyone, especially those with joint issues or orthopedic concerns. If jogging or running is too intense, consider incorporating intervals

of jogging or running into your walking routine.

- **Stair Climbing:** Climbing stairs is an excellent weight-bearing exercise that engages multiple muscle groups, including the legs, hips, and glutes. It also provides a cardiovascular workout while strengthening bones in the lower body. If you don't have access to stairs, you can use a stair climber machine at the gym or a step platform at home.
- **Jumping Rope:** Jumping rope is a high-impact weight-bearing exercise that can help improve bone density, especially in the lower body. It also provides a cardiovascular workout and improves coordination and agility. Start with short intervals of jumping rope and gradually increase the duration as your fitness level improves.
- **Dancing:** Dancing, whether it's ballroom, salsa, Zumba, or hip-hop, is a fun and effective weight-bearing exercise that engages the whole body. Dancing involves dynamic movements, changes in direction, and weight shifts, which help stimulate bone growth and improve balance and coordination.
- **Hiking**: Hiking on uneven terrain provides a challenging workout for the lower body and engages stabilizing muscles, which can help improve bone density and strength. Plus, being outdoors in nature offers additional mental health benefits.
- **Strength Training with Weights:** Strength training exercises using free weights, resistance bands, or weight machines can also be effective for improving bone health. Exercises like squats, lunges, deadlifts, and overhead presses target major muscle groups and stimulate bone growth. Make sure to use proper form and start with lighter weights before progressing to heavier loads.
- **Osteostrong:** This new technology which emulates high impact loading, was invented to reverse Osteoporosis but it's overall strengthening can't be beat. While the studies are still accumulating, with a major one under peer review right now, the anecdotal evidence with

DEXA confirmed improvements is extensive. Strength, power and balance are rapidly improved with this technology as well.

- **Plyometric Exercises:** Plyometric exercises, such as jump squats, box jumps, and burpees, involve explosive movements that increase force on the bones and stimulate bone remodeling. These high impact exercises are high risk for injury; however, and should be performed with caution and under the supervision of a qualified fitness professional, especially for individuals with joint issues or orthopedic concerns.

When incorporating weight-bearing exercises into your routine, it's important to choose activities that you enjoy and feel comfortable doing. Start gradually and progress slowly to avoid injury. Consider a personal trainer or choose activities with an instructor or a coach. If you have any existing health conditions or concerns, consult with a healthcare provider or fitness professional before beginning a new exercise program.

Strength Training

Strength training is an essential component of a well-rounded exercise routine for bone health. While weight-bearing exercises like walking, jogging, and stair climbing help stimulate bone growth and maintain bone density, strength training specifically targets muscle strength and bone strength. Strength training is beneficial for bone health as training exercises, such as squats, lunges, dead lifts, and presses, involve applying resistance to the bones through muscle contractions. This mechanical stress stimulates bone cells to lay down new bone tissue, leading to increased bone density and strength. Strong muscles support and protect the bones, reducing the risk of fractures and falls. Strength training exercises target major muscle groups, including the legs, hips, back, chest, shoulders, and arms, helping to improve overall muscle strength and function.

Many strength training exercises require stability and balance, which are essential for preventing falls and maintaining mobility. Improving balance and stability through strength training can reduce the risk of falls and fractures, especially in older adults. Strengthening the muscles around the joints helps improve joint stability and reduce the risk of injuries, such as sprains and strains. This is particularly important for individuals with osteoarthritis or other joint-related conditions.

Strength training stimulates bone remodeling, a process by which old or damaged bone tissue is replaced with new, stronger bone tissue. Activities that stress the bones trigger the bone-forming cells to jump into action and lay down new and stronger bone, building boned density over time. This helps maintain bone health and integrity, especially in areas prone to fracture, such as the hips and spine. Strength training increases muscle mass, which can boost metabolism and aid in weight management. Maintaining a healthy weight is important for bone health, as excess body weight can increase stress on the bones and joints. Strength training exercises can be modified to accommodate individual fitness levels, goals, and limitations. Whether using free weights, resistance bands, weight machines, Osteostrong or body weight exercises, there are a variety of options available to suit different preferences and abilities.

To incorporate strength training into your routine for optimal bone health, aim to perform strength training exercises at least two to three times per week. targeting all major muscle groups. Start with lighter weights and gradually increase the resistance as you build strength and confidence. If you are in a market where there is an

Osteostrong franchise, consider their groundbreaking technology for musculoskeletal strength building, a sweat free alternative or add-on to your fitness routine that involves triggering osteogenesis in one short, weekly session. In all strength training activities, it is important to use proper form and technique to minimize the risk of injury. If you're new to strength training or have specific health concerns, consider working with a qualified fitness professional, such as a personal trainer or physical therapist, to develop a safe and effective strength training program tailored to your needs.

Athletes and Bone Health

Athletes rely on strong and healthy bones to support optimal performance and reduce the risk of injuries, especially those related to repetitive stress or high-impact activities. Bone health plays a critical role in athletic performance, as well as in the prevention of fractures, stress fractures, and other bone-related injuries. Here's how bone health relates to athletic performance and injury prevention:

- **Bone Strength and Density:** Athletes with higher bone mineral density (BMD) and bone strength have a reduced risk of fractures and stress fractures, which can sideline them from training and competition. Adequate bone density is essential for absorbing impact forces and withstanding the repetitive loading experienced during athletic activities.
- **Muscle-Bone Interaction:** Strong muscles exert mechanical forces on bones during physical activity, which stimulates bone remodeling and helps maintain bone mass and strength. Athletes who engage in regular weight-bearing and muscle-strengthening exercises promote bone health through this muscle-bone interaction.
- **Nutrition and Calcium Intake:** Proper nutrition, including adequate

calcium and vitamin D intake, is essential for supporting bone health in athletes. Calcium is a key mineral for bone formation and remodeling, while vitamin D facilitates calcium absorption and bone metabolism. Athletes should consume a balanced diet rich in calcium-containing foods and consider supplementation if dietary intake is inadequate.

- **Hormonal Factors:** Hormonal imbalances, such as low estrogen levels in female athletes or low testosterone levels in male athletes, can negatively impact bone health and increase the risk of bone-related injuries. Female athletes with menstrual irregularities or amenorrhea (absence of menstruation) may be at higher risk of osteoporosis and stress fractures due to hormonal disruptions.

- **Energy Availability:** Female athletes participating in sports that emphasize leanness or require weight management may be at risk of low energy availability, which can lead to hormonal disturbances, menstrual dysfunction, and impaired bone health (referred to as the female athlete triad). Low energy availability can compromise bone remodeling and increase the risk of stress fractures.

- **Training Load and Over training:** Excessive training load, rapid increases in training volume or intensity, and inadequate recovery can place excessive stress on bones and increase the risk of overuse injuries, including stress fractures. Athletes should incorporate proper rest, and recovery strategies into their training programs to prevent over training and promote bone health.

- **Biomechanical Factors:** Biomechanical factors such as foot mechanics, running gait, and training surfaces can influence bone loading and stress distribution during athletic activities. Athletes should pay attention to proper footwear, running mechanics, and training techniques to minimize the risk of overuse injuries and optimize bone health.

- **Monitoring and Screening:** Regular monitoring of bone health, including bone density testing and screening for risk factors such as menstrual irregularities, low energy availability, and hormonal imbalances, can help identify athletes at increased risk of bone-related injuries. Early detection and intervention can prevent complications and support optimal bone health and athletic performance.

In summary, athletes should prioritize bone health as an integral component of their training and performance regimen. By adopting strategies to support bone health, including proper nutrition, training load management, biomechanical optimization, and regular monitoring, athletes can reduce the risk of injuries and optimize their athletic potential and longevity in their chosen sport. Working with healthcare providers, sports medicine professionals, and nutrition experts can help athletes develop individualized strategies to promote bone health and performance while minimizing the risk of bone-related injuries.

In closing this chapter, we would like to include a couple functional exercises that can be practices at home to improve mobility, agility and balance. A functional movement pattern is a movement that mimics activities of daily living and engages multiple muscle groups to perform a specific task. Here's an example of a common functional movement pattern:

Squat to Pick Up an Object:

- Stand with your feet hip-width apart, toes pointed slightly outward, and arms hanging by your sides.
- Engage your core muscles and maintain a neutral spine (straight back).
- Bend your knees and lower your hips back and down, as if sitting back into a chair.

- Keep your chest lifted and your weight on your heels as you descend into the squat position.
- Lower yourself until your thighs are parallel to the ground or as far down as comfortable while maintaining proper form.
- Reach forward with your arms to grasp the object you intend to pick up.
- Keep your back straight and your chest lifted as you lift the object by pushing through your heels and straightening your legs.
- Stand up tall, squeezing your glutes at the top of the movement.
- Carry the object close to your body and maintain good posture as you walk or move to your desired location.
- To release the object, reverse the movement pattern by bending your knees and lowering it to the ground with control.

This functional movement pattern, the squat to pick up an object, engages multiple muscle groups, including the quadriceps, hamstrings, glutes, core muscles, and upper body muscles (such as the shoulders and arms). It promotes lower body strength, stability, and mobility while also reinforcing proper lifting mechanics and posture, which are essential for preventing injuries during activities of daily living. Incorporating functional movement patterns like this into your exercise routine can improve overall functional capacity and help maintain independence and quality of life.

Here's another example of a functional movement pattern:

Lunge with Rotation:

- Stand with your feet hip-width apart and arms at your sides.
- Take a step forward with your right foot, bending both knees to lower your body into a lunge position.

- Keep your front knee aligned with your ankle and your back knee hovering just above the ground.
- Engage your core muscles to maintain balance and stability.
- While in the lunge position, rotate your torso to the right, bringing your arms straight out in front of you.
- Return to the starting position by rotating your torso back to the center and pushing through your right heel to stand back up.
- Repeat the lunge with rotation on the opposite side, stepping forward with your left foot and rotating your torso to the left.
- Continue alternating sides for the desired number of repetitions.

This functional movement pattern combines a lower body exercise (the lunge) with a rotational movement of the torso, engaging multiple muscle groups including the quadriceps, hamstrings, glutes, core muscles, and obliques. It promotes lower body strength, balance, coordination, and rotational stability, which are important for activities such as walking, climbing stairs, and twisting while reaching or lifting. Integrating functional movement patterns like the lunge with rotation into your workout routine can improve overall movement quality and functional capacity for daily activities.

Physical activity is one of the most important habits to incorporate into your healthy bones action plan. Start small, just add one thing each day and keep doing it until it is part of your routine. We promise you will feel better right away, both mentally and physically.

8

Balance and Fall Prevention

Fall prevention strategies are essential for reducing the risk of falls and fall-related injuries, especially among older adults. Fractures can be devastating at any age and fall-prevention is fracture prevention. Here are some key fall prevention strategies:

- **Exercise Regularly:** Engaging in regular physical activity helps improve strength, balance, flexibility, and coordination, reducing the risk of falls. Focus on exercises that target balance, such as tai chi, yoga, and balance training exercises, as well as strength training to build muscle strength and stability.
- **Review Medications:** Some medications can increase the risk of falls by causing dizziness, drowsiness, or changes in blood pressure. Review medications with a healthcare provider to identify potential side effects and interactions that may affect balance or cognitive function. Adjustments to medication dosage or timing may be necessary to minimize fall risk.
- **Get Regular Vision and Hearing Checks:** Poor vision and hearing can impair awareness of surroundings and increase the risk of falls. Have regular vision and hearing screenings to detect changes in vision or

hearing that may impact balance and mobility. Wear prescription glasses or hearing aids as needed to improve sensory perception and awareness. If your vision prescription changes, be aware of possible impacts to balance and movement.

- **Ensure Home Safety:** Make modifications to the home environment to reduce fall hazards. Install grab bars and handrails in bathrooms and stairways, improve lighting in hallways and entryways, remove tripping hazards such as loose rugs and clutter, and secure electrical cords and cables out of pathways. Consider using nonslip mats in the bathroom and shower and adding nightlights in key areas. (See Chapter 5)

- **Wear Proper Footwear:** Choose supportive, well-fitting footwear with nonskid soles to provide stability and traction while walking. Avoid wearing shoes with high heels, slippery soles, or loose straps that can increase the risk of slips and falls. Invest in a pair of good hiking boots, maybe two, one for spring and summer and one for fall and winter, with good ankle support and souls that grip appropriately make all the difference while hiking and give the wearer more confidence against falls.

- **Use Assistive Devices:** If mobility or balance is compromised, use assistive devices such as canes, walkers, or mobility aids to provide support and stability while walking. Ensure that assistive devices are properly fitted and in good condition to maximize effectiveness and safety. Even if you do not use an assistive device for activities of daily living, consider a walking stick or trekking pole as an added safety measure against falls when walking or hiking.

- **Be Mindful of Environmental Factors:** Be aware of environmental factors that may increase the risk of falls, such as uneven or slippery surfaces, changes in elevation, poor lighting, or obstacles in walkways. Take precautions to navigate safely in unfamiliar or hazardous environments, and use caution when walking on wet or icy surfaces.

- **Stay Hydrated and Well-Nourished:** Dehydration and poor nutrition can contribute to weakness, fatigue, and impaired cognitive function, increasing the risk of falls. Drink plenty of water to stay hydrated, and maintain a balanced diet rich in nutrients to support overall health and mobility.
- **Practice Safe Behaviors:** Be mindful of safe behaviors to prevent falls, such as taking your time when getting up from a seated or lying position, using handrails when climbing stairs, and avoiding risky behaviors such as standing on unstable surfaces or using a chair to retrieve objects that are out of reach.
- **Stay Active and Engaged:** Remaining socially active and engaged in meaningful activities can help maintain physical and cognitive function, reducing the risk of falls and promoting overall well-being. Stay connected with friends and family, participate in community activities, and engage in hobbies or interests that promote movement and mental stimulation.

By implementing these fall prevention strategies, individuals can reduce the risk of falls and injuries, maintain independence, and enjoy a higher quality of life, especially as they age. It's important to assess individual fall risk factors and tailor prevention strategies to address specific needs and challenges. Consulting with a healthcare provider or occupational therapist can help develop a personalized fall prevention plan based on individual circumstances and preferences.

The Costs of Falls

Falls can have significant economic implications due to healthcare costs, loss of productivity, mental health, and long-term care expenses. Here are some key points regarding the cost of falls:

- **Healthcare Costs:** Falls often result in injuries that require medical attention, hospitalization, and rehabilitation. The direct medical costs associated with falls include emergency department visits, hospital stays, surgeries, medications, diagnostic tests, and out-patient rehabilitation services. These healthcare expenses can be substantial, especially for older adults who may experience more severe injuries and complications from falls.
- **Long-Term Care:** Falls can lead to long-term disability and functional decline, requiring ongoing care and assistance with activities of daily living. Individuals who experience falls may require long-term care services, such as home health care, assisted living, or nursing home placement, which can incur significant costs over time. The need for long-term care following a fall can also place financial strain on families and caregivers.
- **Loss of Productivity:** Falls can result in temporary or permanent disability, leading to a loss of productivity in the workforce. Individuals who are injured in falls may need to take time off work or retire early due to disability, resulting in lost wages and reduced earning potential. Employers may also experience decreased productivity and increased healthcare costs related to falls among employees.
- **Quality of Life:** Falls can have a profound impact on an individual's quality of life, independence, and well-being. Older adults who experience falls may fear falling again, leading to activity restriction, social isolation, and decreased participation in community and leisure activities. The psychological and emotional toll of falls can contribute to depression, anxiety, and decreased overall satisfaction with life.
- **Healthcare Utilization:** Falls often lead to multiple healthcare encounters, including visits to emergency departments, primary care providers, specialists, and rehabilitation facilities. The increased healthcare utilization associated with falls can strain healthcare sys-

tems and resources, leading to longer wait times, higher healthcare costs, and decreased access to care for other patients.

- **Preventive Measures:** Investing in fall prevention strategies and interventions can help reduce the economic burden of falls by preventing injuries, hospitalizations, and long-term care admissions. Cost-effective fall prevention programs, home modifications, community-based initiatives, and clinical interventions can help mitigate fall risk and reduce healthcare costs associated with falls.

In summary, falls impose significant economic costs on individuals, families, healthcare systems, and society as a whole. By implementing effective fall prevention measures and addressing modifiable risk factors, we can help reduce the financial burden of falls and improve outcomes for individuals at risk of falling. Investing in fall prevention is not only cost-effective but also essential for promoting healthy aging, preserving independence, and enhancing quality of life for older adults.

9

The Future

Children and their future bone health

There are growing concerns about the potential impact of today's children's bone health on their future as seniors. Several factors contribute to these concerns: Sedentary lifestyles, increased screen time, and decreased physical activity among children may negatively affect bone development and density. Insufficient weight-bearing exercise and poor dietary habits, including low calcium intake and high consumption of processed foods, can compromise bone health during childhood and adolescence, crucial times in bone development which determine future bone health and resilience. Inadequate intake of essential nutrients such as calcium, vitamin D, protein, and micronutrients during childhood and adolescence can impair bone development and increase the risk of osteoporosis later in life. Poor dietary habits and reliance on processed or convenience foods may contribute to nutritional deficiencies among children and adolescents.

Childhood and adolescence are critical periods for bone development, with peak bone mass typically reached by early adulthood. Factors that influence bone health during these formative years, such as genetics, growth hormone levels, hormonal changes, and lifestyle behaviors, can have unsuspecting long-lasting effects on bone strength and density. Increased use of electronic devices and sedentary behaviors that accompany those activities, may reduce opportunities for weight-bearing exercise and physical activity, which are essential for optimal bone health, especially in these years of maximum bone building opportunity. Prolonged sitting and screen time may also displace outdoor play and other activities that promote bone development and muscle strength.

Additionally the rising prevalence of childhood obesity is a major concern for bone health, as excess body weight can place additional stress on developing bones and increase the risk of musculoskeletal problems. Childhood obesity is associated with metabolic disturbances, inflammation, and hormonal imbalances that may impact bone metabolism and contribute to lower bone density, all contributing or perhaps more accurately, taking away from future bone health and increasing future fracture risk.

There is a need for increased awareness and education about the importance of bone health during childhood and adolescence. Promoting healthy lifestyle habits, encouraging physical activity, and providing access to nutritious foods can help support optimal bone development and lay the foundation for lifelong bone health. The alternative is not a pretty one. Poor bone health during childhood and adolescence can have long-term consequences, including increased risk of fractures, osteoporosis, and related complications in later life. Addressing bone health concerns early in life can help mitigate these risks and promote healthy aging in adulthood and beyond.

Childhood and adolescence are critical periods for bone development, with peak bone mass typically achieved by mid to late teens. Maximizing peak bone mass during these formative years is essential for reducing the risk of osteoporosis and fractures later in life. While osteoporosis is often associated with older adults, fractures also occur in children and adolescents, particularly during periods of rapid growth and physical activity. According to the Centers for Disease Control and Prevention (CDC), approximately 1 in 3 children will experience a fracture before reaching adulthood. Worldwide, there is growing recognition of the importance of addressing childhood bone health. According to the International Osteoporosis Foundation (IOF), osteoporosis and low bone mass are estimated to affect over 200 million children and adolescents globally. Without intervention, this trend may contribute to a significant burden of osteoporosis-related fractures in the future. We do wish to acknowledge that socioeconomic factors including access to healthcare and environmental influences can impact children's bone health outcomes. Disparities in bone health exist among different populations, with marginalized communities often facing higher rates of nutritional deficiencies, physical inactivity, and other risk factors for poor bone health.

Addressing bone health concerns during childhood and adolescence presents opportunities for prevention and intervention. Promoting healthy lifestyle habits, including regular physical activity, balanced nutrition, adequate sun exposure, and access to healthcare, can help support optimal bone development and reduce the risk of future fractures. By prioritizing bone health promotion during childhood and adolescence, we can help children build strong and resilient bones that support lifelong health and well-being. In summary, addressing concerns about children's bone health is important for maximizing peak bone mass, reducing the risk of fractures, and promoting lifelong skeletal health.

By prioritizing bone health promotion efforts early in life, we can help children build strong and resilient bones that support their health and well-being into adulthood and beyond.

The Future of Bone Health for Everyone

Nothing is changing faster than medicine, healthcare and our understanding of wellness and longevity. As history has shown us, life gets better. So we look forward to improvements in understanding and recognizing the importance of this subject with regard to our overall healthspan and quality of life. As we look to the future of bone health, there are several key areas that hold promise for advancements and improvements:

- **Personalized Medicine:** The future of bone health will likely involve more personalized approaches to prevention, diagnosis, and treatment. Advances in genetics, biomarkers, and technology may enable healthcare providers to tailor interventions to individuals' specific risk factors, genetic predispositions, and lifestyle factors.
- **Precision Nutrition:** Nutrition plays a crucial role in bone health, and future research may uncover more about how specific nutrients, dietary patterns, and personalized nutrition strategies can optimize bone density and strength. Precision nutrition approaches may help individuals achieve optimal bone health outcomes based on their unique nutritional needs and preferences.
- **Innovative Therapies:** Emerging therapies, including novel medications, biologics, gene therapies, and regenerative medicine approaches, hold promise for improving bone health outcomes and reducing fracture risk. Research into new treatments for osteoporosis, bone regeneration, and musculoskeletal disorders may lead to more effective and targeted interventions.

- **Technology and Digital Health:** Digital health technologies, such as wearable devices, mobile apps, telemedicine platforms, and remote monitoring tools, have the potential to revolutionize how bone health is managed and monitored. These technologies may facilitate early detection of bone health issues, enhance patient engagement, and improve access to care.
- **Preventive Strategies:** The future of bone health will likely place greater emphasis on preventive strategies, including lifestyle interventions, community-based programs, and public health initiatives aimed at reducing modifiable risk factors for fractures. Proactive measures to promote bone health from childhood through older adulthood may help prevent fractures and improve overall population health.
- **Interdisciplinary Collaboration:** Collaboration among healthcare providers, researchers, policymakers, educators, and community stakeholders will be essential for addressing the multifaceted nature of bone health. Interdisciplinary approaches that integrate medical, nutritional, behavioral, and environmental factors will be key to achieving optimal bone health outcomes across the lifespan.
- **Health Equity and Access:** Ensuring equitable access to bone health resources, screening, and treatments will be critical for addressing disparities in bone health outcomes among different populations. Efforts to promote health equity and reduce barriers to care will be essential for improving bone health outcomes for all individuals, regardless of socioeconomic status, race, ethnicity, or geographic location.

Overall, the future of bone health holds promise for advancements in many areas. By embracing these opportunities and working together to prioritize bone health, we can strive to reduce the burden of fractures, improve quality of life, and promote healthy aging for individuals in our communities and worldwide.

10

Resources

Resources

There are several community resources and support options available for individuals seeking to improve and maintain bone health. These resources can provide education, guidance, and opportunities for physical activity, as well as support networks for those dealing with bone-related conditions. Your best way to locate these organizations is through an online search that will deliver local options for you. These suggestions are examples of places to start:

- **Senior Centers:** Many communities have senior centers that offer a variety of programs and services aimed at promoting health and well-being among older adults. Senior centers may offer exercise classes, educational workshops on bone health, nutrition programs, and social activities that encourage active lifestyles and social engagement.
- **Community Centers:** Community centers often host fitness classes, wellness programs, and recreational activities that promote physical activity and overall health. Seniors and other community members

can participate in activities such as walking clubs, yoga classes, strength training programs, and balance and fall prevention workshops.

- **Public Libraries:** Public libraries may offer resources such as books, videos, and online databases that provide information on bone health, osteoporosis prevention, and healthy aging. Libraries may also host educational seminars or guest speakers who discuss topics related to bone health and wellness.
- **Local Hospitals and Health Clinics:** Hospitals and health clinics may offer bone density screenings, health fairs, and educational events focused on bone health and osteoporosis prevention. Healthcare providers and specialists may also provide community outreach programs, support groups, and resources for individuals with osteoporosis or other bone-related conditions.
- **Fitness Facilities:** Gyms, fitness centers, and recreation facilities often offer exercise programs and classes specifically designed to improve bone health, strength, and balance. Group fitness classes, personal training sessions, and aquatic exercise programs may be available for individuals of all ages and fitness levels.
- **Nonprofit Organizations:** Nonprofit organizations dedicated to bone health and osteoporosis awareness may provide resources, support services, and advocacy efforts to raise awareness and promote preventive measures. These organizations may offer educational materials, online forums, support groups, and community outreach programs to help individuals manage bone-related conditions and live healthier lives.
- **Local Parks and Recreation Departments:** Parks and recreation departments may organize outdoor activities, walking groups, and community events that promote physical activity and healthy lifestyles. Seniors and other community members can take advantage of walking trails, fitness equipment, and recreational

facilities in local parks to stay active and maintain bone health.

- **Health Education Programs:** Health education programs offered by community organizations, universities, and healthcare providers may include workshops, seminars, and classes on topics such as osteoporosis prevention, bone-healthy nutrition, fall prevention, and exercise for bone health. These programs provide valuable information and resources to help individuals make informed decisions about their bone health and well-being.

By tapping into these community resources and support options, individuals can access valuable information, services, and opportunities to improve and maintain their bone health, reduce the risk of fractures and falls, and enhance overall quality of life. Collaboration among community stakeholders, healthcare providers, and local organizations can help promote bone health awareness and create supportive environments that facilitate healthy aging for all members of the community.

Additionally, there are numerous online resources available to support individuals interested in learning more about bone health, osteoporosis prevention, and related topics. Some of reputable online resources include:

- **National Osteoporosis Foundation (NOF):** The National Osteoporosis Foundation is a leading nonprofit organization dedicated to promoting bone health and preventing osteoporosis. Their website (www.nof.org) offers a wealth of information on bone health, osteoporosis risk factors, prevention strategies, treatment options, and support resources. The NOF website also features educational materials, interactive tools, and online support communities for individuals affected by osteoporosis.
- **American Bone Health:** American Bone Health is a nonprofit

organization focused on empowering individuals to take control of their bone health through education and advocacy. Their website (www.americanbonehealth.org) provides comprehensive information on bone health, osteoporosis prevention, exercise recommendations, nutrition tips, and fracture prevention strategies. Visitors can access educational articles, videos, and resources tailored to different age groups and risk factors.

- **National Institute of Arthritis and Musculoskeletal and Skin Diseases** (NIAMS): NIAMS, part of the National Institutes of Health (NIH), offers evidence-based information on bone health, osteoporosis, and related musculoskeletal conditions. Their website (www.niams.nih.gov) features educational materials, fact sheets, research updates, and resources for patients and healthcare professionals. Visitors can explore topics such as bone density testing, calcium and vitamin D recommendations, and exercise for bone health.

- **MedlinePlus: MedlinePlus**, a service of the National Library of Medicine, provides reliable health information for consumers and healthcare professionals. Their website (medlineplus.gov) offers a variety of resources on bone health, osteoporosis, fractures, and related conditions. Visitors can access articles, videos, interactive tutorials, and links to reputable organizations and government agencies for additional information and support.

- **WebMD:** WebMD is a popular health information website that covers a wide range of topics, including bone health and osteoporosis. Their Bone Health & Osteoporosis section (www.webmd.com/osteoporosis) provides articles, slideshows, videos, and interactive tools to help individuals learn about risk factors, prevention strategies, treatment options, and lifestyle recommendations for maintaining strong and healthy bones.

- **Mayo Clinic:** The Mayo Clinic website (www.mayoclinic.org) offers extensive information on bone health, osteoporosis, and fracture prevention. Visitors can access articles, patient care guides, videos, and expert insights from Mayo Clinic healthcare professionals. The website covers topics such as bone density testing, calcium and vitamin D supplementation, exercise guidelines, and fall prevention strategies.

These online resources provide valuable information, tools, and support for individuals interested in learning more about bone health, osteoporosis prevention, and strategies for maintaining strong and healthy bones throughout life. It's important to seek information from reputable sources and consult with healthcare professionals for personalized guidance and advice tailored to individual needs and circumstances.

For individuals interested in functional medicine, which focuses on addressing the root causes of health issues and promoting overall wellness through a holistic and personalized approach. Here are a few reputable online resources for functional medicine:

- **Institute for Functional Medicine (IFM):** The Institute for Functional Medicine is a global leader in functional medicine education, training, and research. Their website (www.ifm.org) offers a variety of resources, including educational articles, webinars, podcasts, and online courses for healthcare professionals and the general public. IFM also provides a searchable database of functional medicine practitioners and offers certification programs for healthcare providers.
- **Functional Medicine University (FMU):** Functional Medicine University is an online educational platform that offers courses, webinars, and certification programs in functional medicine. Their website (www.functionalmedicineuniversity.com) provides access to a wealth of educational resources on topics such as nutrition, gut

health, hormone balance, detoxification, and integrative approaches to chronic disease management.

- **The Functional Medicine Blog:** The Functional Medicine Blog, hosted by Chris Kresser, a licensed acupuncturist and functional medicine practitioner, provides evidence-based articles, podcasts, and resources on functional medicine and ancestral health. The blog covers a wide range of topics, including diet and lifestyle interventions, gut health, autoimmune conditions, and personalized approaches to health and wellness.

- **Dr. Mark Hyman:** Dr. Mark Hyman is a prominent functional medicine physician, bestselling author, and educator known for his work in integrative and holistic health. His website (www.drhyman.com) features articles, videos, podcasts, and online programs that focus on functional medicine principles, including personalized nutrition, metabolic health, brain health, and environmental medicine.

- **Functional Medicine Coaching Academy (FMCA):** The Functional Medicine Coaching Academy offers online training and certification programs for health coaches specializing in functional medicine. Their website (www.functionalmedicinecoaching.org) provides information about their curriculum, faculty, and resources for aspiring health coaches interested in applying functional medicine principles to support client wellness.

- **The Dr. Axe Website:** Dr. Josh Axe is a doctor of natural medicine, chiropractor, and clinical nutritionist who advocates for a functional medicine approach to health and wellness. His website (www.draxe.com) offers articles, recipes, supplements, and educational resources on topics such as gut health, hormone balance, immune support, and natural remedies.

These online resources provide valuable information, education, and support for individuals interested in functional medicine and integrative approaches to health and wellness. Whether you're seeking information for personal health management or professional development, these resources can help you learn more about functional medicine principles and strategies for optimizing health and vitality.

Support groups can be invaluable resources for individuals dealing with health challenges, including those related to bone health, osteoporosis, and other musculoskeletal conditions. These groups provide opportunities for individuals to connect with others who share similar experiences, offer emotional support, share information and resources, and learn coping strategies for managing their condition. Here are some options for finding support groups related to bone health:

- **National Osteoporosis Foundation (NOF):** The National Osteoporosis Foundation offers online support communities where individuals affected by osteoporosis and related bone conditions can connect with others, share experiences, and find encouragement and support. These communities provide a safe and supportive environment for asking questions, sharing concerns, and accessing resources on bone health.
- **Local Hospitals and Health Clinics:** Many hospitals and health clinics offer support groups for individuals with osteoporosis, fractures, and other musculoskeletal conditions. These groups may meet in person or virtually and provide opportunities for education, peer support, and social interaction. Check with your local healthcare providers or hospital for information on support groups in your area.
- **Online Forums and Social Media Groups:** There are numerous online forums and social media groups dedicated to bone health, osteoporosis, and related topics. These platforms allow individuals to connect with others worldwide, share experiences, ask questions,

and access information and resources. Websites such as Inspire (www.inspire.com) and PatientsLikeMe (www.patientslikeme.com) offer online communities where individuals can find support and camaraderie.

· **Meetup Groups:** Meetup.com is a platform that connects people with common interests, including health and wellness. You can search for local meetup groups related to bone health, osteoporosis, exercise, or healthy aging in your area. Meetup groups provide opportunities for face-to-face interaction, group activities, and social support within your community.

· **Senior Centers and Community Centers:** Senior centers and community centers often host support groups and wellness programs for older adults, including those dealing with bone health issues. These groups may focus on topics such as osteoporosis prevention, fall prevention, exercise for bone health, and coping strategies for living with chronic conditions. Contact your local senior center or community center for information on available programs and support groups.

· **Nonprofit Organizations:** Nonprofit organizations dedicated to bone health, osteoporosis awareness, and musculoskeletal conditions may offer support groups and peer-to-peer programs for individuals affected by these conditions. These organizations may provide educational materials, online forums, and local support group networks to help individuals connect and share experiences.

By participating in support groups and connecting with others who understand their experiences, individuals dealing with bone health challenges can find comfort, encouragement, and practical advice for managing their condition and improving their quality of life. Whether online or in person, support groups offer valuable opportunities for emotional support, social connection, and empowerment on the journey toward better bone health. The opportunity to connect with someone who can truly understand what you are going through can be an invaluable asset during challenging times. Once you come through your challenge, you can help others navigate their own rough waters.

Finally, a word of encouragement dear reader. This guide was written to help you and everything in it is there for your benefit and education. You are in-charge of your health and healthcare. First and foremost it is the decisions you make on a daily basis that make all the difference in your long term wellness or 'healthspan', a term that recalls the old saying "In the end, it's not the years in your life that count, it's the life in your years." A child born today in the developed world may well live to 100 with the advances in medicine and technology. Independence, mobility, cognitive health, and the ability to live a long and pain-free life is everyone's #lifegoal. Maintaining the foundation of your health, the skeletal system is a smart move towards these goals.

11

Citations

National Institute of Health. (2004) US Department of Health and Human Services. Office of the Surgeon General *Bone Health and Osteoporosis: A Report of the Surgeon General.* . https://www.ncbi.nlm.nih.gov/books/NBK45504/

International Journal of Womens Health (2014, May) *Advances in evaluating the fetal skeleton.* Ann-Edwidge Noel and Richard N. Brown https://www.ncbi.nlm.nih.gov/pmc/articles/PMC4027851/#:~:text=T he%20clavicle%2C%20mandible%2C%20ileum%2C,ossified%20by% 2012%E2%80%9316%20weeks.

Journal of Bone and Mineral Research. (1995 May); *Peak bone mass in young women.* Teegarden D, et al. https://pubmed.ncbi.nlm.nih.gov /7639106/#:~:text=By%20age%2022.1%20%2B%2F%2D%202.5,of% 20peak%20BMC%20is%20attained.

Journal of Clinical Densitometry. (2016, April) *Peak bone mass and patterns of change in total bone mineral density and bone mineral contents from childhood into adulthood.* Juan Lin, MD M.PH., Ph.D, and Yongyun

Shin, Ph.D. et al. https://www.ncbi.nlm.nih.gov/pmc/articles/PMC440 2109/

National Institute of Health. National Institute of Arthritis and Musculoskeletal and Skin Diseases. Bone Mineral Tests: *What the Numbers Mean* https://www.niams.nih.gov/health-topics/bone-mineral-density-tests-what-numbers-mean#:~:text=A%20bone%20mineral%20density%20(BMD,we%20develop%20certain%20medical%20conditions.

National Spine Health Foundation. (2020, May) *Lifelong Nutrition for Healthy Bones* https://spinehealth.org/article/lifelong-nutrition-for-healthy-bones/#:~:text=Physical%20activity%20and%20nutrition%20are,negatively%20affect%20peak%20bone%20mass.

Critical Review Food Science and Nutrition. (2006) *The role of nutrients in bone health, from A to Z.* Christina Palacious https://pubmed.ncbi.nlm.nih.gov/17092827/#:~:text=The%20process%20of%20bone%20formation,D%2C%20potassium%2C%20and%20fluoride.

Journal of Osteoporosis. (2017, Dec) *Nutritional Aspects of Bone Health and Fracture Healing*
Athanasios Karpouzos, Evangelos Diamantis et al. https://www.ncbi.nlm.nih.gov/pmc/articles/PMC5804294/#:~:text=Insufficient%20intake%20of%20certain%20vitamins,healing%20in%20case%20of%20fracture.

John's Hopkins Medicine. *Calcium Supplements Should You Take Them?* https://www.hopkinsmedicine.org/health/wellness-and-prevention/calcium-supplements-should-you-take-them#:~:text=On%20the%20other%20hand%2C%20recent,of%20calcium%20and%20other%20substances.

UCI Health. *Live Well What Smoking Does to Your Bones* https://www.ucihealth.org/blog/2018/11/smoking-bone-health#:~:text=Smoking%20reduces%20the%20blood%20supply,cellular%20functions%20and%20bone%20health.

Alcohol Health and Research World. (1998) *Alcohol's Harmful Effects to the Bone* H. Wayne Sampson, Ph.D https://www.ncbi.nlm.nih.gov/pmc/articles/PMC6761900/#:~:text=Alcohol's%20action%20on%20young%2C%20growing,are%20more%20susceptible%20to%20fracture.

Journal of Endocrinology. (2000, Aug) *Role of genetic factors in the pathogenesis of osteoporosis* T L Stewart et al https://pubmed.ncbi.nlm.nih.gov/10927613/#:~:text=Osteoporosis%20is%20a%20polygenic%20disorder,mutations%20in%20a%20single%20gene.

American Journal of Geriatric Psychiatry. (2020 June). US Department of Veterans Affairs. *Hoarding Disorders in Older Adulthood* Catherine R. Ayers Ph.D https://www.ncbi.nlm.nih.gov/pmc/articles/PMC7295124/

National Institute of Health. National Institute on Aging. *Falls and Fractures in Older Adults: Causes and Prevention* https://www.nia.nih.gov/health/falls-and-falls-prevention/falls-and-fractures-older-adults-causes-and-prevention#:~:text=Foot%20problems%20that%20cause%20pain,likely%20you%20are%20to%20fall.

WebMD. *Vitamin K* R. Morgan Griffin https://www.webmd.com/vitamins-and-supplements/supplement-guide-vitamin-k

www.ingramcontent.com/pod-product-compliance
Lightning Source LLC
Chambersburg PA
CBHW051834250726

48659CB00005B/1837